CONTENTS

PREFACE

Before we begin let's set the stage with a remark.
Menopause is a phase, in a women life that brings about
challenges well as opportunities for growth and self-care
renewal. There is a misunderstanding and lack of conversation
around menopause despite its widespread occurrence that often
leads to confusion or worry. Many women feel alone during this
journey as they face symptoms and struggle to find guidance on
confidently navigating these changes, with vitality and vigor.
This Complete Guide, to Health and Well-being with a focus
on Hormonal Balance is designed to change the way people
see things about this topic. This detailed and caring guide
helps women prepare for menopause by providing them with
knowledge and useful techniques. By discussing areas such, as
nutrition, the importance of exercise taking care of emotions,
hormonal balance and more this handbook supports women
in enhancing their well-being during this stage of life.
Each part shares information based on understanding and real-
world experience to provide helpful and practical solutions,
for managing typical menopausal signs and symptoms
effectively and naturally. You will discover advice on dealing
with flashes improving the quality of sleep; maintaining
the health of bones and heart; and nurturing mental well-
being and emotional strength. Furthermore the book
explores the overlooked connections between menopause
and aspects such, as wellness, stress handling and lifestyle
changes that can ease the transition period and set the
stage for a fulfilling and healthy post-menopausal life.
This book offers more, than health tips.
It's a campaign for self-care and empowerment. It is designed

to help readers make informed decisions about their own well-being. and face this stage of life with purpose and strength. Let Thrive Through menopause serve as your guide as you discover that menopause is more than just a time to be endured. But it was a powerful moment of change. which with the right tools It can lead to renewed vigor, balance and vitality. This is blossoming through menopause—health care. health and recovery

INTRODUCTION

Menopause is a natural and transformative chapter of life, bringing a variety of changes and new experiences. While it may present its own set of challenges, it also offers a meaningful opportunity for growth, self-discovery, and understanding your body on a deeper level. This book is crafted to accompany you through this transition, offering practical guidance, compassionate insights, and a focus on whole-body wellness to help you thrive.

As your body adapts to hormonal shifts, focusing on physical, mental, and emotional well-being can help you navigate these changes with greater ease. Embracing balanced nutrition, regular physical activity, stress reduction, and self-care practices can support you in feeling resilient, energized, and empowered throughout this stage and beyond. Achieving hormonal balance is key to navigating menopause with confidence. As hormone levels such as estrogen, progesterone, and testosterone fluctuate, they can influence mood, energy, sleep, and metabolism. By making mindful lifestyle choices and considering natural or medical therapies, when necessary, you can create a foundation for balance and wellness. This book provides you with insights into maintaining hormonal health, allowing you to approach menopause as a time of renewal and strength

CHAPTER 1

This chapter explores the main elements of the menopausal cycle. It explains clearly and simply what women face. Common symptoms and the important role of hormones in this process. Our goal is to give you a complete understanding of what to expect during this life transition. This makes menstruation more convenient and less scary.

UNDERSTANDING MENOPAUSE:

Menopause is the event in a woman's life that ends her reproductive years. It usually occurs between ages 45 and 55, although it may occur earlier or later in some people. But menopause is officially recognized when a woman has not had a period for 12 consecutive months - - - this signifies the cessation of menstruation and loss of fertility. Although menopause comes with a variety of symptoms and physical changes, But it is very important to know that this is not a disease or medical condition. Rather, it is a normal part of the aging process that affects all women.

MENOPAUSE PROGRESSION:

From perimenopause to menopause:
Menopause is a gradual process. Appears periodically Instead it happened suddenly. Being aware of these steps allows women to predict and prepare for the changes involved.

• Menopause (Transition period):
This first stage, which begins several years before actual menopause. It is characterized by a gradual decrease in estrogen production in the ovaries and fluctuating hormone levels. Women may experience irregular menstrual cycles and symptoms of early menopause, such as hot flashes and mood swings. and sleep is disturbed There are various greatly over the past several years

*** Menopause (cessation of menstruation):**
A woman enters menopause when she has not had a period for 12 months. At this point, The release of ovaries has stopped. And estrogen levels dropped significantly. This stage marks the end of a woman's reproductive years and may be followed by more serious symptoms due to the sharp rejection in hormone production.

• post menopause (years after menopause):
This phase opens the period after menopause. Some serious symptoms of menopause may subside as women continue to adjust to lower hormone levels. During this time It is important to focus on maintaining health. This is because the long-term effects of reducing estrogen may increase the risk of diseases such as osteoporosis and cardiovascular disease.

HORMONAL CHANGES DURING MENOPAUSE:

The main cause of physical and emotional changes during menopause is hormonal fluctuations. The main hormones involved in this process are estrogen, progesterone, and testosterone.

• Estrogen:
Estrogen is extremely important in regulating the female reproductive system. Including menstruation and fertility. When women enter menopause Estrogen levels will begin to decrease. This drop in estrogen triggers common symptoms of menopause, such as hot flashes and noticeable sweating. and vaginal dryness

• Progesterone:
Progesterone acts with estrogen to regulate the menstrual cycle. When estrogen levels decrease Progesterone also decreases. As a result, menstruation is irregular during menopause. After menstruation completely stops Progesterone levels will remain low.

• Testosterone:
Embora is usually associated with men. Testosterone is also important for women's health. Helps maintain muscle mass, libido, and energy levels. during menopause Testosterone levels can also decrease. This results in decreased sexual desire and feelings of fatigue.

These hormonal changes affect the body. Causes many symptoms When hormone levels fluctuate The body will try to adjust. This explains why symptoms can continue or become more severe.

CHAPTER 2

EXPLORING HORMONAL RESEARCH

This section delves into the scientific aspects of hormone balancing. and explores essential hormones that have a major impact on women's health during menopause. When understanding these hormones and their functions Readers will gain insight into the causes of specific symptoms. and learn strategies for improving hormonal health. We also explore thyroid and kidney function. The impact of hormonal imbalance on general well-being and the importance of hormone testing in managing menopausal symptoms.

RESEARCH ON ESTROGEN, PROGESTERONE, AND TESTOSTERONE:

The three hormones are estrogen, progesterone, and testosterone. It is essential for women's reproductive health and general well-being. When entering menopause These hormones begin to fluctuate. It reveals the many physical and emotional changes that women go through.

• Estrogen:

Estrogen is the main female hormone that controls the menstrual cycle and reproductive system. It also helps maintain healthy blood, skin, and cardiovascular system function. During the period near menopause Estrogen levels are not safe. This results in irregular periods and normal menopausal symptoms such as heartburn. night sweats and vaginal dryness as menopause progresses Estrogen levels are significantly reduced. This leads to long-term effects, such as an increased risk of osteoporosis and heart disease.

• Progesterone:

Progesterone works with estrogen to regulate the menstrual cycle and prepare the body for pregnancy. In the years before menopause As the year progresses, progesterone decreases as semen ejaculates less. A decrease in hormones can cause symptoms such as mood swings, irritability, and anxiety.

Progesterone also plays a mediating role. tone. Lower testosterone levels can also impact mood and cognitive function, resulting in what some women describe as "brain fog."
Collectively, these hormones maintain a delicate equilibrium in a woman's body. When one or more become imbalanced, it can trigger a range of symptoms affecting physical, emotional, and mental well-being.

THE IMPORTANCE OF THE THYROID AND ADRENAL GLANDS

In addition to the sex hormones (estrogen, progesterone, and testosterone), two other important glands play an important role in maintaining hormonal balance during menopause. Including the thyroid and adrenal glands...

Thyroid gland:

The thyroid gland in the neck secretes thyroid hormones (T3 and T4) and controls the body's metabolism, energy, and temperature. Hormonal changes during menopause can increase the sensitivity of the thyroid gland. This may result in weight gain. fatigue and mood swings Women with hypothyroidism may experience more severe menopausal symptoms, such as chills, dry skin, and hair loss. Proper thyroid function is important to overall health. This is especially true during the hormonal changes of menopause.

Adrenal glands:

The adrenal glands, located on top of the kidneys, produce stress hormones such as cortisol and adrenaline. This is because estrogen production in the ovaries decreases during menopause. The adrenal glands compensate by producing small amounts of estrogen to maintain balance. However, chronic stress can cause the adrenal glands to become overworked. It places more emphasis on cortisol production than estrogen. This may aggravate menopausal symptoms such as adrenal fatigue, fatigue, and anxiety. and mood swings Effective management of stress during menopause is essential to ensure proper adrenal function and hormonal balance.

EFFECTS OF HORMONAL IMBALANCE ON HEALTH

Hormonal imbalances during menopause can affect many aspects of a woman's well-being. When hormones such as estrogen, progesterone, testosterone is not coordinated. The body will struggle to maintain balance. This results in a number of symptoms and health problems:

Physical health:

Hormonal imbalances can cause a variety of physical symptoms. Including abdominal weight gain, hot flashes, and night sweats. and tired Lack of estrogen can reduce bone density and increase the risk of osteoporosis. Women may experience joint pain and muscle weakness. Low estrogen affects skin health. Leads to dryness, thinness and loss of elasticity.

Emotional and mental health:

Low levels of estrogen and progesterone have a huge impact on your mood and mental well-being. during menopause Many women experience increased anxiety, depression, irritability, and mood swings. Testosterone imbalance can affect cognitive function. This causes difficulty concentrating or "brain fog." Hormone-related sleep disorders can also aggravate emotional and cognitive challenges.

Sexual health:

Low testosterone and estrogen levels can result in decreased libido, vaginal dryness, and discomfort during sex. These changes can affect a woman's feelings of intimacy and sexual confidence. Hormonal imbalances also affect body image. causing nervousness or irritability

Sustainable health results:

Hormonal imbalances can increase the chance of long-term health problems. For example, lower estrogen levels after menopause are associated with a higher chance of heart disease. And a long-term consequence of estrogen deficiency through changes in cholesterol and blood vessel elasticity is osteoporosis, which results from decreased bone density.

Understanding the impact of these imbalances on your physiology is important for managing symptoms and for protecting your long-term well-being during and after menopause.

HORMONE EVALUATION: WHAT YOU WANT TO REALIZE

Hormone trying out serves as a critical technique for detecting and comprehending hormonal imbalances, especially at some stage in menopause. These checks help determine if decreased hormone stages are contributing to signs and might tell remedy selections, starting from life-style modifications to supplements or hormone alternative therapy (HRT).

Hormone Test Varieties:

Hormone ranges may be assessed through various strategies, consisting of:

Timing of Tests:

If you are encountering intense menopausal signs and symptoms including extreme warm flashes, mood fluctuations, or exhaustion, hormone level trying out may be useful. This permits your healthcare provider to create a tailored remedy strategy. Testing is likewise treasured whilst thinking about hormone replacement therapy, as it aids in figuring out appropriate dosages.

Interpreting Test Outcomes:

Hormone test results can monitor whether your estrogen, progesterone, testosterone, or different hormones are insufficient, excessive, or out of balance. For instance, low estrogen tiers might give an explanation for signs and symptoms like vaginal dryness and warm flashes, while inadequate progesterone could make a contribution to insomnia or anxiety. with this information, being in your possession you and your healthcare provider can create a personalized plan to restore hormonal balance and alleviate symptoms.

CHAPTER 3

MEDICAL TREATMENT FOR MENOPAUSE:

Menopause is a natural part of a woman's life. And proper treatment can lead to overall health. strength and balance This chapter delve into strategies for managing menopausal symptoms. Emphasis is placed on eating strategies. exercise and reducing stress Women can relieve symptoms, increase their life expectancy, and improve their overall health by making lifestyle changes.

To Maintain Hormonal Balance, it is Important To:
Eating a healthy diet is important for managing symptoms such as hot flashes, weight gain, and mood swings. and fatigue at the same time, it helps support hormone production and balance.

IMPORTANT FOODS FOR MENOPAUSE:

Some foods are often referred to as "Superfoods" are especially beneficial during the menstrual cycle. This is because it is high in nutrients which support hormone regulation and create symptom control. Incorporating the following into one's diet One can have major effects on health:

- **Flax seeds:** These seeds contain lignans. This is a hormone-like substance that can help reduce inflammation and improve hormonal balance. It's also high in fiber and omega-3s, which are beneficial for heart health.
- **Green leafy vegetables:** Vegetables such as spinach, kale, and broccoli are high in calcium and magnesium. It is beneficial to bone health and reduces the risk of osteoporosis. This is a common concern during menopause.
- **Berries:** Fruits like blueberries, strawberries, and strawberries contain high levels of antioxidants that help fight oxidative stress. which is a substance that can make menopausal symptoms worse It also supports cognitive function and elevates mood.
- **Soybeans:** Phytoestrogens are found in soybeans. This is a plant that mimics hormones in the body. This includes foods that contain soy, such as tofu, tempeh, and eda

. **Fatty Fish:** Salmon, mackerel, and sardines are rich in omega-3 fatty acids, which help reduce inflammation, support brain health, and improve mood during menopause.

Incorporating these beneficial foods into one's weight loss program can help alleviate signs and symptoms whilst boosting electricity, mood, and normal fitness during menopause.

NUTRITION FOR HORMONAL IMBALANCE

During menopause, certain nutrients become increasingly more critical due to hormonal modifications. Deficiencies in those nutrients can exacerbate menopause signs or result in long-time period fitness troubles. Key vitamins to take note of encompass:

Calcium: With declining estrogen ranges, women face an improved threat of osteoporosis. Ensuring ok calcium consumption (through foods like dairy products, leafy greens, and fortified plant milks) is vital for keeping bone health.

Vitamin D: This diet works along with calcium to preserve strong bones. Many ladies are deficient on this nutrient, particularly in regions with constrained daylight. Consider taking a supplement or consuming foods like fortified dairy merchandise, fish, and eggs.

Magnesium: is a essential mineral that promotes relaxation, enhances sleep nice, and helps bone health. Insufficient magnesium can result in muscle spasms, sleeplessness, and emotions of unease. Nuts like almonds, leafy greens which include spinach, and seeds like pumpkin are terrific resources of magnesium.

The B vitamin family, especially B6, B12, and folate, plays a vital role in maintaining energy levels, regulating mood, and supporting cognitive function. These vitamins can help alleviate fatigue and mental fog during menopause. Whole grains, eggs, and legumes are rich in B vitamins.

Iron deficiency may occur in some women during perimenopause due to irregular or heavy menstrual cycles. This mineral is essential for energy production and preventing anemia. Incorporate lean meats, legumes, and dark green leafy vegetables into your diet to ensure adequate iron intake.

Focusing on these nutrients during menopause can help optimize bodily functions, reduce symptoms, and prevent potential health complications in the future.

SUPPLEMENTAL SUPPORT FOR HORMONAL BALANCE:

In conjunction with a nutritious diet, certain supplements can offer additional assistance in managing menopausal symptoms and maintaining hormonal equilibrium. Some of the most effective supplements for menopause include:

- **Black Cohosh:** This traditional herbal remedy has been utilized for generations to alleviate hot flashes, night sweats, and mood fluctuations.
- **Vitamin D and Calcium:** These nutrients are critical for maintaining bone health and reducing osteoporosis risk, particularly as estrogen levels decline.
- **Omega-3 Fatty Acids:** These supplements help decrease inflammation, promote cardiovascular health, and support cognitive function during menopause.**Maca Root:** An adaptogenic herb known for its ability to balance hormones and enhance mood, energy, and libido.

Probiotics: Maintaining gut health during menopause is important because of its impact on hormone regulation. Probiotic supplements help maintain a healthy digestive system and balance the digestive system. Although dietary supplements are helpful But it is important to seek advice from a health professional to ensure that the products are suitable for your individual needs...

EXERCISE FOR HEALTH AND FITNESS:

Regular exercise is one of the most effective strategies for managing menopausal symptoms and improving your overall health. Exercise helps balance hormones. Maintain a healthy weight, improve mood, and increase energy levels. This is because the metabolism slows down during menopause. It is important to include a variety of exercises to maintain strength and cardiovascular fitness.

BENEFITS OF RESISTANCE TRAINING AND AEROBIC EXERCISE:

• Resistance training:
Strength training during menopause is important because it helps prevent loss of muscle mass and bone density. When estrogen levels decrease Women are therefore at greater risk of osteoporosis and muscle weakness. Lifting weights or doing resistance exercises can help build and maintain muscle mass. Strengthen your bones and improve metabolism Exercises like squats, lunges, and push-ups are great for strengthening your core and lower body muscles.

• Aerobic exercise:
Cardiovascular activities such as walking, jogging, cycling or swimming promote heart health. Helps control body weight and reduce the severity of hot flashes Aerobic exercise improves blood circulation. Make your heart strong and help manage stress At least 30 minutes of moderate aerobic exercise most days of the week can greatly improve your energy and overall well-being.

Both resistance training and aerobic exercise are important for preserving muscle strength, bone density, and heart health during menopause.

ENHANCING FLEXIBILITY AND RELAXATION THROUGH YOGA AND PILATES

Yoga:
During menopause, yoga serves as an terrific approach for boosting flexibility, reducing pressure, and fostering relaxation. The combination of breathing sports and subtle moves in yoga can help mitigate tension, enhance mood, and doubtlessly reduce the frequency of hot flashes. Stretching-focused poses focused on the hips, spine, and shoulders can alleviate anxiety and raise circulate. Moreover, yoga cultivates mindfulness and emotional equilibrium, that are specifically positive at some point of the emotional fluctuations related to menopause.

Pilates:
Pilates emphasizes growing core power, enhancing posture, and growing flexibility. This mild workout form is specifically beneficial for menopausal women because it strengthens the pelvic floor, belly muscle tissues, and lower again - regions typically suffering from hormonal shifts. Additionally, Pilates aids in enhancing balance and coordination, thereby reducing the

chance of falls related to declining bone density.

Both yoga and Pilates not handiest make contributions to physical properly-being but also provide a feel of tranquility and intellectual clarity, supporting ladies in managing stress and maintaining emotional balance during menopause.

By concentrating on right nutrition, supplementation, and consistent bodily activity, women can certainly manage menopausal signs and decorate their common health. This chapter offers steering for ladies to take rate of their properly-being via trustworthy, green, and sustainable lifestyle adjustments that sell hormonal stability, power, and relaxation.

CHAPTER 4

NAVIGATING MENOPAUSE SYMPTOMS WITH NATURAL REMEDIES

As menopause unfolds, it could deliver plenty of signs and symptoms that could have an effect on each day life. Understanding these shifts and exploring natural approaches to control them could make this degree of existence snugger. This chapter highlights a number of the maximum commonplace signs of menopause and affords realistic tactics to ease the transition, from techniques for hot flashes to recommendations for keeping wholesome pores and skin.

COOLING STRATEGIES FOR HOT FLASHES AND NIGHT SWEATS

Hot flashes: night time sweats are common and frequently challenging symptoms of menopause, marked via sudden warm temperature and excessive sweating which could disrupt sleep and day by day comfort.

•**Staying Cool**: Wearing mild, breathable fabric, using a fan, and making use of cooling gel packs can all help modify frame temperature.

• **Hydrate:** Staying hydrated with the aid of ingesting cold water all through the day may additionally help lessen the frequency of warm flashes.

• **Herbal Remedies:** Some girls discover comfort from supplements like black cohosh or nighttime primrose oil. It's satisfactory to consult a healthcare professional earlier than beginning any natural remedies.Mood Swings and Emotional Well-being

Hormonal changes during the menstrual cycle can cause mood swings such as anger, sadness, or anxiety. Maintaining emotional health is essential to everyone's well-being.

• **Mindfulness and Meditation:** Mindfulness or meditation techniques can help to calm the mind. relieve stress and stabilize the mood

• **Exercise for endorphins:** Exercise such as walking, swimming, or yoga releases endorphins. which is a natural mood regulator

• **Herbal supplements:** Herbs such as St. John's wort. John's wort can help balance your mood. But always consult a health professional for advice.

IMPROVING SLEEP QUALITY AMID SLEEP DISTURBANCES

Sleep troubles are not unusual all through menopause, frequently because of night time sweats, tension, or hormonal changes.

• **Create a Restful Environment:** Set up a cool, quiet, and darkish room. Blackout curtains and retaining the temperature round 65°F (18°C) can beautify sleep high-quality.

• **Natural Sleep Aids:** Supplements like melatonin and valerian root may additionally guide **relaxation and resource restful sleep.**

• **Sleep Routine:** Going to bed and waking up on the identical time each day allows alter sleep styles.

MANAGING WEIGHT GAIN AND METABOLISM CHANGES

Menopause can effect metabolism, every now and then making it less complicated to advantage weight, specially across the stomach. Maintaining a healthful weight can assist enhance electricity and save you different health problems.

• Balanced Diet: Prioritize a food regimen wealthy in lean proteins, complete grains, and a number of fruits and greens. Limiting processed ingredients and delicate sugars also can assist manipulate weight.

• Strength and Cardio Training: Resistance sporting activities build muscle and boom metabolism, even as sports like on foot and biking assist burn calories.

• Mindful Eating: Paying attention to hunger cues and practicing portion manipulate can help prevent overeating. Supporting Hair, Skin, and Nail Health During Menopause

Hormonal shifts can result in modifications in hair, skin, and nails, frequently resulting in dryness or thinning.

• Hydrate and Nourish: Drinking enough water and ingesting healthy fat, including those located in avocados, nuts, and salmon, can promote moisture and resilience in hair and skin.

• Biotin and Collagen Supplements: These vitamins can support nail energy, hair texture, and skin elasticity

• Use of Natural Oils: Applying oils like argan or jojoba to skin and hair may additionally assist with dryness, enhancing texture and appearance.

CHAPTER 5

MENTAL HEALTH AND EMOTIONAL WELL-BEING

Menopause changes go beyond physical changes. This includes important emotional adjustments. Hormonal fluctuations during this time can have a profound effect on a woman's mental state. This often results in mood swings. feeling of anxiety and depressive symptoms This chapter delves into the psychological effects of menopause. Provides techniques for maintaining mental balance social networks to promote emotional resilience During this life The value of stress reduction methods is also emphasized.

PSYCHOLOGICAL EFFECTS OF MENOPAUSE

Menopause brings about a number of physiological changes that can trigger a wide range of emotional reactions. Some women view it as the final stage of their lives. This can lead to feelings of sadness, depression, or anxiety. Other people may experience a sense of independence as they pass through puberty. Although each person's emotional response will vary, but common psychological symptoms during menopause include:
The emotional landscape of menopause can be further shaped by concurrent life events, such as adult children leaving home. (Empty Nest Syndrome) Changes in personal relationships. or career transition...

DEALING WITH ANXIETY AND DEPRESSION:

Although emotional problems are more prevalent during menopause, but there are effective strategies for dealing with anxiety and depression. Identifying the signs and using coping mechanisms can help women deal with this emotion more smoothly.

CONSULT A MENTAL HEALTH PROFESSIONAL:

Consultation with a mental health professional is important for severe or long-lasting symptoms of anxiety or depression. Therapy, especially cognitive behavioral therapy (CBT), can help women change negative thought patterns. Manage stress and develop more effective coping strategies...

Physical Activity:
Exercise has been proven to alleviate anxiety and melancholy. It stimulates the production of endorphins—herbal temper enhancers—and aids in pressure reduction. Engaging in regular aerobic workout, power education, and practices like yoga can make a contribution to advanced emotional properly-being all through menopause.

Healthy Lifestyle Practices:
Dietary and way of life selections play a great function in mental health control. Reducing alcohol and caffeine intake, retaining a balanced diet rich in omega-3 fatty acids and antioxidants, and ensuring adequate sleep can assist stabilize temper and mitigate symptoms of anxiety and depression.

Developing Mindfulness and Stress Management Techniques
Mindfulness involves being fully present and engaged within the moment, that can assist reduce stress and promote emotional equilibrium. During menopause, mindfulness practices can be

especially useful in dealing with temper fluctuations, anxiety, and emotions of crush.

Conscious Breathing:

Practicing deep, intentional respiration can help calm the worried gadget and alleviate feelings of tension. Dedicating a couple of minutes every day to attention on slow, managed breaths can decrease stress hormones like cortisol and foster a feel of rest.

Mindfulness Practices:

Quieting the thoughts thru meditation enables women to enhance their emotional recognition. Dedicating 10 to 15 minutes daily to meditative practices can cause reduced tension, improved concentration, and improved emotional stability.

Progressive muscle relaxation includes alternately contracting and enjoyable various muscle agencies, which aids in alleviating physical tension and minimizing pressure. This method is in particular useful for dealing with sleeplessness or aggravating mind. Maintaining a magazine serves as a amazing method for emotional expression and strain remedy. By documenting their thoughts and feelings, girls can manner emotions, discover styles, and brainstorm capability answers to their challenges.

Developing a addiction of gratitude can redirect awareness from terrible emotions and foster a extra constructive outlook. Daily reflection on things to be pleased about can beautify typical emotional nicely-being.

These mindfulness strategies can function effective gear for strain reduction and emotional equilibrium at some stage in menopause.

THE SIGNIFICANCE OF SOCIAL CONNECTIONS AND COMMUNITY

During menopause, having a guide system comprising buddies, family, or a community of ladies experiencing similar changes is crucial. Feeling related and supported can mitigate feelings of isolation and enhance emotional resilience.

Loved Ones:

Transparent verbal exchange with pals and circle of relatives can offer necessary emotional support in the course of tough intervals. Sharing experiences and feelings with others enables normalize menopausal feelings and cultivates a sense of belonging.

Support Networks:

Many ladies locate solace in menopause support businesses, in which they are able to trade reviews, benefit insights from others, and construct a community. Online forums and local gatherings provide safe areas to speak about signs and symptoms, answers, and emotional challenges.

Professional Assistance:

If emotional difficulties end up overwhelming, searching for assist from a therapist or counselor can offer precious insights and coping strategies. Professional steerage can help ladies in navigating complicated feelings and growing methods to manage stress, anxiety, or melancholy.

Community Engagement:

Participating in activities consisting of volunteering, attending social occasions, or becoming a member of organization exercise instructions can offer a feel of purpose and connection. Community involvement allows fight loneliness and gives opportunities to shape new relationships for the duration of this transitional lifestyles segment.

The emotional adventure via menopause may be tumultuous at times, however by way of fostering strong social connections and using sensible pressure control strategies, women can navigate this lifestyles degree with greater self-belief and serenity.

CHAPTER 6

INTIMATE RELATIONSHIPS AND REPRODUCTIVE WELLNESS

The menopausal transition can significantly affect a woman's intimate life and reproductive fitness. These alterations regularly stem from hormonal fluctuations affecting sexual drive, responsiveness, and vaginal wellness. However, it is totally possible to sustain a fulfilling and healthy intercourse life in the course of and after menopause. This chapter explores common shifts in reproductive wellbeing, practical remedies for discomfort, and techniques to foster closeness along with your sizable other.

SHIFTS IN SEXUAL DESIRE AND RESPONSIVENESS:

A primary challenge for the duration of menopause is the alteration in sexual appetite or desire. Many ladies notice a decline in sexual interest, which may be attributed to both hormonal shifts and emotional factors. Physical responses at some stage in intimate encounters may additionally trade.

It's vital to recognize that changes in sexual preference vary significantly among individuals. While some women revel in reduced libido, others won't locate any changes, and some would possibly even experience a renewed feel of sexual liberation.

TACKLING VAGINAL DRYNESS AND DISCOMFORT:

Vaginal dryness ranks most of the maximum typical bodily symptoms of menopause and can result in soreness at some point of sex. As estrogen levels decline, the vaginal tissues end up thinner, much less bendy, and drier, potentially making sexual pastime uncomfortable or maybe painful. Fortunately, numerous effective answers exist for dealing with these signs.

Vaginal Moisturizers: These over-the-counter merchandises are designed for ordinary use to maintain hydration in vaginal tissues. Consistent application of vaginal moisturizers can help alleviate dryness and decorate comfort.

Lubricants: During sexual activity, using water-based or silicone-based totally lubricants can reduce friction and discomfort. It's important to pick out a lubricant free from irritants or fragrances that would purpose similarly infection.

Vaginal Estrogen: Some ladies advantage from low-dose vaginal estrogen, available as lotions, rings, or pills. This treatment facilitates repair moisture and elasticity to the vaginal tissues by way of handing over estrogen directly to the region without affecting the entire frame.

Pelvic Floor Exercises: Strengthening the pelvic floor muscular tissues through Kegel exercises can enhance blood circulate to the pelvic location and decorate sexual sensation. This can also deal with problems like urinary incontinence, which can affect sexual

confidence.
Addressing vaginal dryness is vital for keeping comfort and leisure throughout sexual activity, and those solutions can assist alleviate soreness even as selling better reproductive health.

COMMUNICATING WITH YOUR PARTNER: NURTURING INTIMACY:

Open and honest speak is important for preserving intimacy in the course of menopause. Changes in libido, body belief, and sexual responsiveness can occasionally create distance in a courting if no longer addressed overtly. Discussing your desires, concerns, and goals together with your accomplice can assist both of you navigate this transition with empathy and know-how.

Communicate Your Experience:

Share together with your partner how menopause is impacting your physical and emotional nation. Open communique can help prevent misunderstandings and fortify your emotional bond. Discuss your options all through intimate moments, together with the need for extended foreplay or gentler techniques.

Embrace Non-Sexual Intimacy:

Remember that physical closeness is not confined to intercourse. Embracing, smooching, interlocking hands, and different affectionate gestures can hold intimacy. Exploring various types of closeness can alleviate overall performance anxiety and help each people feel cherished and preferred.

Practice Adaptability:

Both companions need to exercise endurance as they adapt to

new patterns of intimacy. Sexual encounters can also require greater time and talk, however being open to novel ways of bodily connection can lead to deeper emotional bonds.

Seek professional help:

If communication or intimacy is a problem A therapist or relationship counselor can provide helpful support and advice. Therapy can address any emotional or relational challenges that arise during this transition. Ultimately, this strengthens the partnership.

Effective communication promotes an environment in which both partners can communicate their needs. and work together to maintain a satisfying close relationship.

STRATEGIES FOR MAINTAINING SEXUAL WELLNESS

Menopause doesn't sign the quilt of a pleasing intercourse existence—pretty the alternative! With suitable changes, many ladies maintain to enjoy a dynamic and healthy sexual courting throughout and after menopause. Consider these techniques to hold the passion alive:

Emphasize Self-Care: Maintaining your bodily and emotional properly-being is vital for sexual fitness. A balanced diet, normal workout, adequate sleep, and powerful strain management all make a contribution to stepped forward sexual health and power.

Plan Intimate Moments: While spontaneity may additionally lower with age and changing instances, intimacy would not ought to lessen. Setting aside everyday time for "date nights" or intimate encounters can assist hold the relationship and ensure each partners prioritize their dating.

Explore New Experiences: Sexual relationships evolve, and menopause can be an opportune time to find out new methods of connecting. This would possibly involve experimenting with distinctive styles of touch, incorporating intercourse aids, attempting function-playing, or altering your routine. Embracing new experiences can re-light excitement and desire.

Consult Healthcare Professionals: If sexual discomfort persists or libido troubles extensively impact your quality of existence, searching for recommendation from a healthcare company. In addition to vaginal estrogen, medical doctors may recommend different remedies such as testosterone dietary supplements or medicines specifically designed to enhance sexual choice in girls.

Mindfulness and Relaxation: Being present and aware at some point of intimate moments can enhance both emotional and bodily bonds. By concentrating at the contemporary enjoy and savoring the sensations of bodily touch and intimacy, couples can gain a stronger connection and heightened amusement.

Sexual health performs a essential role in overall fitness, and whilst approached accurately, the menopausal phase can provide an possibility for rejuvenation and more profound intimacy among partners.

CHAPTER 7

SKELETAL HEALTH DURING THE MENOPAUSAL TRANSITION:

Menopause increases the importance of a woman's skeletal health. When estrogen levels decrease Bones will become more brittle. As a result, there is an increased chance of osteoporosis and bone fractures. This chapter explores the relationship between menopause and bone health. How to maintain strong bones and how to prevent fractures and joint discomfort. Understanding how to nourish your skeletal system during menopause can help you maintain an active, healthy lifestyle for longer.

WEAK POINTS OF OSTEOPOROSIS IN POSTMENOPAUSAL WOMEN:

Osteoporosis is characterized by brittle bones that are easily at risk of breaking. This is a major concern for postmenopausal women because estrogen drops dramatically. Which is an important hormone for maintaining bone density during this life...

FACTORS THAT INCREASE THE RISK OF OSTEOPOROSIS DURING MENOPAUSE:

Estrogen is essential for new bone formation. Facilitates the absorption of calcium and the formation of new bone cells. Low estrogen levels during menopause lead to a faster rate of bone breakdown. and slows down the formation of new bone This imbalance can result in rapid loss of bone density. Increases women's risk of osteoporosis and bone fractures.

Prevalence of Osteoporosis:

Studies imply that about 1 in three ladies over 50 will enjoy osteoporosis-associated fractures. The backbone, hips, and wrists are in particular prone, and these fractures can notably impact mobility and nice of existence.

Acknowledging the heightened risk of osteoporosis all through menopause is essential for prevention and control. Fortunately, there are effective strategies to shield and make stronger your bones.

INCREASE BONE STRENGTH AND DURABILITY:

Keeping your bones strong is important to prevent osteoporosis throughout and after menopause. There are several effective ways to promote bone health:

Nutrition:
Your nutritional choices play a critical position in preserving bone fitness. Consuming nutrient-wealthy meals excessive in calcium, nutrition D, and magnesium can help bone strength. Include leafy vegetables, dairy merchandise, almonds, and fortified plant-based milks for your every day meals. Ensuring a nicely-balanced weight loss program with suitable nutrients is vital for bone regeneration.

Weight-Bearing Physical Activity:
Exercise is one of the maximum robust approaches to preserve and enhance bone density. Weight-bearing sports which include taking walks, walking, dancing, and hiking stimulate bone boom by means of applying strain to the bones. Resistance sporting events like weightlifting or using resistance bands also build muscle and decorate bone electricity. These sports can assist mitigate the charge of bone loss for the duration of menopause.

Flexibility and Balance Training:
Activities that beautify flexibility and balance, which includes yoga and tai chi, are also essential. They assist lessen fall threat through enhancing coordination and balance, which becomes

increasingly vital as you age.

Avoid Tobacco and Excessive Alcohol Consumption:
Smoking and excessive alcohol consumption can weaken bones and accelerate bone loss. Quitting smoking and restricting alcohol consumption can significantly decrease your threat of osteoporosis.

By integrating these lifestyle practices into your ordinary, you may construct and hold bone strength and reduce the risk of osteoporosis.

CALCIUM, VITAMIN D, AND EXERCISE: THEIR IMPACT ON BONE HEALTH

Specific vitamins and physical sports are crucial for preserving bone energy at some stage in menopause. We'll look at how calcium, diet D, and constant exercise make contributions to extra sturdy bones.

Calcium:

As the inspiration of healthful bones, calcium will become an increasing number of crucial during menopause while the frame's calcium absorption decreases. Women elderly 50 and above have to devour no less than 1,200mg of calcium every day. This may be done thru dairy products, fortified foods, or calcium dietary supplements if necessary.

Vitamin D:

Facilitating calcium absorption and selling bone development, nutrition D is vital. Even a calcium-rich weight loss plan can be insufficient to prevent bone loss without adequate nutrition D. Sources encompass solar publicity, certain ingredients along with fatty fish, and dietary supplements. Postmenopausal girls are counseled to devour six hundred to 800 IU of vitamin D each day.

Exercise:

Physical interest is similarly critical as nutrients for bone fitness.

Weight-bearing sporting activities pressure bones and stimulate bone formation. Regular exercise now not best continues bone density however also strengthens muscle mass, supporting bones and decreasing the risk of falls and fractures.

Combining a calcium-wealthy eating regimen, sufficient vitamin D consumption, and everyday exercise can successfully guard bones during menopause.

MITIGATING FRACTURES AND JOINT DISCOMFORT

As bones weaken at some point of menopause, stopping fractures and addressing joint ache turns into vital. Osteoporosis increases fracture threat, at the same time as hormonal changes can affect joint tissues, main to ache and stiffness. Here are strategies to minimize those risks

Preventing Falls:

Falls are a number one motive of fractures in older adults. Ensure domestic safety by using disposing of tripping hazards, installing rest room snatch bars, and the use of non-slip mats. Regular balance exercises, consisting of yoga, can enhance balance and decrease fall probability.

Managing Joint Pain:

Menopausal hormonal modifications can purpose inflammation and joint ache. Maintain joint fitness via ordinary exercising, stretching, and weight control. Consider low-effect sporting events like swimming or Pilates to alleviate joint ache without excessive strain.

Bone Density Scans:

A bone density scan (DEXA experiment) measures bone mineral density and assesses fracture risk. Women over sixty five, or younger with osteoporosis danger elements, need to undergo bone density checking out. Based on effects, docs may also advocate preventive treatments, which includes medicinal drugs or lifestyle adjustments.

Medications:

In a few times, medicines may be essential to save you or treat osteoporosis. Bisphosphonates, hormone remedy, and different capsules can sluggish bone loss and decrease fracture threat. Implementing these techniques can substantially lessen the danger of fractures and joint pain at some point of and after menopause, promoting healthful bones and joints.

CHAPTER 8

HEART DISEASE DURING MENOPAUSE

The menopausal transition is an important time in a woman's life. with changes in heart health Although heart disease is the leading cause of death among women, But the risk increases after menopause due to hormonal fluctuations. especially low estrogen This chapter delves into the impact of menopause on heart health, important factors such as cholesterol and blood pressure. and strategies for improving heart health through nutrition, exercise and reducing inflammation, you name it.

Linking menopause and heart health:
Menopause causes drastic hormonal changes in a woman's body. Most notable of these is a decrease in estrogen levels. Estrogen plays a protective role in the cardiovascular system. And a lack of estrogen results in an increased risk of heart disease.

Effects of menopause on the heart:
Estrogen plays a role in making blood vessels flexible. Promotes healthy cholesterol levels and increase blood circulation The decrease in estrogen after menopause can result in hardening of the arteries and increased cholesterol levels. Both of which result in an increased risk of heart disease. and more than that Metabolic changes can cause weight gain. and increases the chance of heart problems

Timing of Increased Risk:
The chance of coronary heart sickness doesn't right away spike at the onset of menopause however step by step increases in the

subsequent years. Women have to be in particular vigilant about their coronary heart fitness at some stage in perimenopause (the transitional phase main to menopause) and beyond.

Recognizing the connection between menopause and cardiovascular health is vital for implementing preventive measures and retaining heart wellness as you age.

CHOLESTEROL, BLOOD PRESSURE, AND HEART DISEASE

Cholesterol:

Menopause can trigger an growth in LDL (terrible) cholesterol and a lower in HDL (good) cholesterol. Elevated LDL ldl cholesterol can cause arterial plaque accumulation, narrowing blood vessels and increasing the chance of coronary heart attacks and strokes. Regular cholesterol monitoring is important, mainly after menopause, to make sure tiers stay inside a wholesome range.

Blood Pressure:

Blood stress often rises with age, however menopause can boost up this manner. As estrogen degrees decline, blood vessels may lose elasticity, impeding blood drift. This can bring about high blood pressure (high blood pressure), a enormous risk element for heart disease and stroke.

Heart Disease:

Menopause elevates the danger of atherosclerosis, the hardening of arteries due to plaque buildup. This can result in heart disorder, the maximum typical purpose of dying among postmenopausal women. Symptoms of heart ailment in girls might also vary from the ones in men, which include extra diffused symptoms like fatigue, shortness of breath, and again ache as opposed to simply chest pain.

Tracking those elements is critical to maintaining cardiovascular health throughout menopause and beyond. Regular consultations with your healthcare issuer can help you stay informed about capacity risks and stay on top of your schedule.

Promote cardiovascular health through nutrition and exercise.

It is important to embrace a happy lifestyle to protect your cardiovascular system during menopause. Proper nutrition and regular exercise are fundamental to maintaining a healthy and adaptable heart.

Nutrition strategies for heart health:

Heart-friendly foods can help control cholesterol, blood pressure, and weight. which is an important factor in reducing the risk of heart disease The required formula is:

Focus on whole grains: Whole grains like oats, quinoa, and brown rice are high in fiber, which helps lower cholesterol.

Beneficial fats: To fight inflammation and support heart function. Include heart-protective fats like omega-3s, which are found in fish, flaxseeds, and nuts. Swap out saturated and trans fats for healthier alternatives like olive oil and avocado.

Abundant Produce: Fruits and greens are wealthy in antioxidants, fiber, and essential nutrients that bolster typical health and shield the heart.

Minimize Sodium and Processed Foods: High sodium intake can raise blood strain. Reducing processed ingredients, regularly excessive in delivered salt, sugar, and unhealthy fats, is vital for coronary heart health.

PHYSICAL ACTIVITY FOR CARDIAC FITNESS

Consistent exercise is paramount for heart energy. It helps decrease cholesterol, improve blood stress, and hold a wholesome weight. Strive for as a minimum one hundred fifty mins of moderate exercise weekly. Beneficial alternatives include:

Aerobic Activities: Walking, swimming, biking, and dancing correctly elevate coronary heart fee and decorate cardiovascular fitness.

Resistance Training: Weight lifting or the use of resistance bands builds muscle, reduces body fat, and helps heart fitness. It additionally allows prevent osteoporosis, a common menopausal challenge.

Flexibility and Balance Workouts: Yoga and Pilates now not only improve flexibility and balance but additionally alleviate strain, positively impacting coronary heart fitness.

By integrating a nutritious diet with ordinary bodily activity, you could considerably lower heart sickness danger and hold cardiac health all through menopause and beyond.

MITIGATING INFLAMMATION AND ENHANCING HEART WELLNESS

Inflammation plays a crucial role in coronary heart ailment development, specifically as the body undergoes menopausal changes. Chronic low-grade inflammation can damage blood vessels and contribute to arterial plaque formation. Fortunately, numerous strategies can reduce inflammation and sell heart well being.

Anti-Inflammatory Nutrition:
Incorporating ingredients that combat infection can help heart health. Top choices consist of

Oily Fish: Salmon, mackerel, and sardines are considerable in omega-three fatty acids, regarded to lessen inflammation and decrease heart disorder hazard.

Berries: Blueberries, strawberries, and raspberries are packed with antioxidants that combat irritation.

Dark Leafy Greens: Spinach, kale, and collard greens are wealthy in vitamins and minerals that lower oxidative stress and irritation.

Nuts and Seeds: Almonds, chia seeds, and flaxseeds offer wholesome fat and fiber that assist cardiac health.

Managing Stress:
Persistent pressure can raise irritation and adversely affect cardiovascular health. Embracing stress-reduction practices which include mindfulness, managed breathing, and stretching sporting

activities can aid in reducing pressure, lowering inflammation, and enhancing universal fitness.

Sleep Quality:

Insufficient sleep can boost inflammation levels and negatively effect heart health. Strive for 7-8 hours of restful sleep nightly to enable bodily repair and recovery. Establishing a calming pre-sleep ordinary and addressing sleep disruptions (like hot flashes or night time sweats) throughout menopause is important for heart wellbeing.

Abstaining from Tobacco and Limiting Alcohol:

Smoking and excessive alcohol use are sizable danger elements for coronary heart disease. Ceasing tobacco use and limiting alcohol consumption to slight quantities (one drink day by day for girls) can drastically lessen irritation and safeguard the coronary heart.

By focusing on minimizing irritation through nutritional choices, way of life adjustments, and pressure control, you may similarly improve your cardiovascular fitness all through menopause.

CHAPTER 9

DIGESTIVE HEALTH AND MENOPAUSE

Digestive health is crucial for typical nicely-being, and for the duration of menopause, it becomes even more critical. Hormonal shifts can have an impact on the digestive machine, and an unbalanced intestine microbiome may, in flip, affect hormone tiers. This bankruptcy will discover how menopause impacts digestion, the significance of the gut microbiome in hormonal equilibrium, and the advantages of probiotics, prebiotics, and dietary changes for maintaining a wholesome digestive machine.

THE IMPACT OF HORMONAL CHANGES ON DIGESTION:

Menopause brings approximately big hormonal fluctuations that could affect nearly each bodily device, consisting of digestion. Estrogen and progesterone tiers differ and decline, influencing intestine characteristic in numerous approaches:

Decelerated Digestion:

Reduced estrogen and progesterone stages can slow down the digestive technique, ensuing in signs such as bloating, constipation, and well known discomfort. Many girls word changes in bowel behavior and enjoy indigestion greater often at some stage in menopause.

Increased Bloating and Gas:

Hormonal shifts can also cause extra frequent bloating and gas. This may be due to the slower movement of food through the digestive tract, that can purpose extended fermentation of undigested meals via intestine bacteria, resulting in gas and bloating.

Digestive Sensations:

Hormonal fluctuations during menopause also cause sensitivities to certain foods. Some women discover that they are more sensitive to foods that may not have caused problems in the past, such as dairy or gluten.

Being aware of these digestive changes can help make adjustments to support better digestive happiness and overall well-being during menopause.

EFFECTS OF GUT MICROBES ON HORMONAL BALANCE

The digestive system consists of a large community of bacteria and microorganisms. These are collectively known as the gut microbiome. This is important for overall health and hormonal balance. Sometimes called the "second brain," this ecosystem interacts with many body systems and can affect estrogen levels during menopause.

The Estrobolome's Function:

A precise subset of gut bacteria, termed the estrobolome, is chargeable for metabolizing and regulating estrogen. These microorganisms produce enzymes that have an impact on estrogen interest and help preserve right hormonal stability. Disruptions in gut fitness can affect estrogen metabolism, doubtlessly exacerbating menopausal signs and symptoms.

Effects on Inflammation and Emotional State:

The gut microbiome additionally performs a function in regulating irritation and temper, both of that can effect menopausal symptoms. For instance, intestine bacteria contribute to the manufacturing of neurotransmitters like serotonin, which impacts mood and stress responses. Maintaining a nicely-balanced microbiome can as a result assist emotional properly-being and doubtlessly alleviate menopause-associated anxiety or irritability.

ENHANCING HORMONAL HEALTH THROUGH MICROBIOME MANAGEMENT

Supporting the intestine microbiome thru dietary and way of life selections can resource in hormone law. This consists of eating ingredients excessive in fiber, probiotics, and prebiotics, which sell the growth of useful microorganism.

By fostering a healthy intestine microbiome, individuals can assist hormonal equilibrium and potentially lessen menopausal signs.

Digestive Wellness: The Role of Probiotics, Prebiotics, and a Nutritious Diet

Maintaining intestine fitness during menopause includes consuming a balanced eating regimen wealthy in probiotics, prebiotics, and other nutrients that support the digestive machine. Let's have a look at how these additives contribute to a healthier gut.

Probiotics and Gut Health:

Probiotics are beneficial bacteria that may enhance the balance of microorganisms in the gut. They are observed in fermented ingredients which include yogurt, kefir, sauerkraut, kimchi, and miso. Probiotics resource digestion, help save you bloating and constipation, and can contribute to reducing irritation.

Selecting Appropriate Probiotics:
Probiotic dietary supplements are to be had and may be custom designed to cope with specific wishes. Look for strains like Lactobacillus and Bifidobacterium, that are recognized to aid digestion and average intestine fitness.
Prebiotics as Nourishment for Beneficial Bacteria:
Prebiotics are varieties of fiber that serve as food for useful gut bacteria. They are found in ingredients which include garlic, onions, bananas, asparagus, and oats. Prebiotics sell the increase and thriving of useful microorganism, supporting the estrobolome and helping keep a balanced gut microbiome.
Incorporating Prebiotics into Your Diet:
Including plenty of prebiotic-rich meals for each day meals can help maintain a numerous and robust gut bacteria population, helping digestion and hormonal fitness.
High-Fiber Diet for Digestive Health:
Fiber is vital for ordinary digestion and basic gut health. An eating regimen considerable in fruits, vegetables, entire grains, nuts, and seeds offers the important fiber to preserve a wholesome digestive device. Fiber aids in regulating bowel moves, helps healthful blood sugar levels, and nourishes beneficial gut bacteria.
Fiber Categories:
Both dissoluble and indissoluble fibers serve important capabilities. Dissoluble fiber, found in ingredients together with oatmeal and apple, can usefully resource in blood sugar regulation. Indissoluble fiber, observed in whole-grain products and greens, assists in shifting meals thru the digestive tract, promoting everyday bowel moves.
The Role of Water in Digestion:
Proper hydration is vital for effective digestion. Water aids in food breakdown and ensures clean functioning of the digestive system. Consuming adequate water for the duration of the day is particularly essential for preventing constipation, a not unusual menopausal trouble because of slowed digestion.
Reducing Intake of Refined Foods and Sugar:
Refined meals and further sugars can negatively affect intestine fitness by way of encouraging the growth of harmful microorganisms and increasing inflammation. Minimizing intake

of these ingredients can assist keep a wholesome microbial balance and assist progressed digestion.

Incorporating probiotics, prebiotics, fiber, and proper hydration into your day-by-day regimen can foster wholesome digestive surroundings that helps both gut health and hormonal equilibrium.

CHAPTER 10

Adjust your lifestyle to flourish during menopause.
Menopause is a major life change. And the lifestyle choices you make during this time can have a huge impact on your experience. By adopting healthy habits Reduce environmental toxins, relax, and focus on personal development. You can cope with menopause in a way that improves your physical health. overall well-being and emotional resilience This chapter delves into how purposeful lifestyle changes can empower you. Towards excellence in menopause and into the future

CREATE HEALTHY ROUTINES AND SELF-CARE STRATEGIES

Cultivating a foundation of healthy habits is important in managing the physical and emotional effects of menopause. Self-care routines can relieve symptoms. Increase life force and makes you more focused Some helpful practices include:

Morning ritual for balance: Starting the day with a simple, focused activity such as stretching, meditation, or a short walk. It will give you a positive attitude for the day ahead. These routines help relieve stress and create calm. This is especially helpful because hormonal changes can increase anxiety.

Mindful Eating and Fluid Intake: Engaging in mindful eating—paying attention to hunger signals. Taste every bite of food and focus on nutrient-dense foods—they can help maintain hormonal balance. Adequate hydration is also important. This is because it can reduce inflammation, remove toxins, and reduce joint discomfort.

Emphasizing Physical Exercise: Regular physical activity not only promotes cardiovascular and skeletal health but can also uplift mood and reduce stress. Strive to incorporate a blend of aerobic, resistance, and flexibility exercises, prioritizing consistency over intensity to maintain a sustainable regimen.

Soothing Evening Practices: Winding down before bedtime with calming pursuits like reading, journaling, or gentle stretching promotes restful sleep, which is essential for effectively managing menopausal symptoms.

Implementing these small yet impactful routines can make a

substantial difference, helping you feel centered and in command during this life phase.

Purifying Your Lifestyle:
 Decreasing exposure to toxins in your environment can reduce the body's stress burden, facilitating better balance during menopause. Environmental toxins can disrupt hormonal health, and making minor adjustments can help safeguard your body.

Household and Personal Care Items: Many common products, from cleaning supplies to beauty items, contain chemicals that can interfere with endocrine function. Choose natural cleaning products and opt for personal care items free of harmful additives such as parabens and phthalates to minimize unnecessary exposure to these chemicals.

Dietary Selections: Consuming organic produce and opting for whole, unprocessed foods can reduce your exposure to pesticides, preservatives, and artificial additives. When possible, select grass-fed or hormone-free meats to further limit intake of synthetic hormones that may interfere with your body's natural balance.

Plastics and Food Storage: Plastics often include BPA and different harmful substances. Transitioning to glass, stainless steel, or ceramic boxes for meals garage can save you these chemicals from seeping into your meals, particularly while using packing containers for heating or storing warm gadgets.

By step by step incorporating those modifications, you create a more fit, toxin-decreased surroundings that supports your body's ability to characteristic optimally.

THE EFFECTIVENESS OF SLEEP, REST, AND RELAXATION FOR WELL-BEING

Sleep plays a critical role in coping with menopausal signs and symptoms, but hormonal fluctuations regularly disrupt sleep patterns. Emphasizing excellent rest and relaxation can enhance resilience and aid physical restoration.

Crafting an Ideal Sleep Environment: Design your bedroom to be cool, dark, and quiet to inspire restful slumber. Consider making an investment in cozy bedding, light-blocking curtains, or ambient noise machines to enhance sleep great.

Maintaining a Regular Sleep Routine: Consistency in bedtime and wake-up times facilitates synchronize your frame's circadian rhythm. Strive for 7-eight hours of nightly sleep to permit for complete physical restoration.

Practicing Mindful Relaxation: Regular engagement in rest physical activities together with deep respiratory, meditation, or modern muscle relaxation can lessen cortisol ranges, result in calmness, and facilitate less complicated sleep onset. Effective sunlight hours stress management can prevent its accumulation and subsequent sleep disturbances.

Utilizing Brief Rests and Power Naps: Short periods of rest or short naps can offer an strength enhance without interfering with nighttime sleep patterns. A 15–20-minute daytime nap may be mainly beneficial for preventing fatigue.

Recognizing relaxation and sleep as important components of

self-care can alleviate menopausal signs and symptoms, sharpen focus, and improve every day functioning.

Personal Development and Accepting Change:

Menopause represents now not only a physical transition but also an opportunity for private and emotional increase. Viewing this section as a danger for self-mirrored image and renewal can foster empowerment and a refreshed experience of reason.

Self-Examination and Aspiration Setting: Use this time to re-examine existence dreams and values, realigning with what's truely important. Establish new personal targets in areas together with health, relationships, profession, or pursuits to domesticate pleasure about destiny possibilities.

Embracing Positive Perspectives on Aging: While menopause may also trigger insecurities about getting old, it is able to additionally be viewed as an opportunity for extended information and self-awareness. Accept physical and emotional adjustments as herbal life progressions, focusing on the strengths and insights that accompany maturity.

Exploring New Interests and Knowledge: Novel studies can spark enthusiasm and motivation. Whether it's adopting a new hobby, growing analyzing behavior, or enrolling in a course, continuous learning and exploration keep intellectual acuity and foster positivity.

Cultivating Support Networks and Community: Maintaining connections with others—be it buddies, own family, or assist organizations—can reduce feelings of isolation in the course of this era. Sharing studies with those present process comparable changes can provide comfort and foster a experience of belonging.

By approaching menopause as an adventure of increase and renewal, this period of change may be transformed into an effective segment of private transformation.

CONCLUSION

EMBRACING YOUR MENOPAUSAL TRANSFORMATION

As you finish this segment, it's essential to acknowledge your increase and resilience. Rather than viewing menopause as a hurdle to overcome, keep in mind it a duration of private development and empowerment. Each step-in knowledge your body's changes and adopting health-aware practices indicates extended self-focus and fortitude. Recognize the tremendous transformation you've gone through and welcome the brand-new possibilities this existence degree gives.

KEY STRATEGIES FOR A WELL-ROUNDED LIFESTYLE

This manual has explored diverse techniques to assist your bodily and intellectual nicely-being at some point of menopause. Key points to recall encompass:

Emphasize Comprehensive Wellness: Recognize the interconnected nature of bodily, emotional, and mental fitness. Nourish your self via balanced nutrients, steady exercising, and effective pressure control strategies.

Support Hormone Balance: Comprehending and keeping hormonal equilibrium can mitigate commonplace menopausal signs and symptoms and make a contribution to long-time period fitness.

Be Attentive to Your Body: Your bodily wishes can also evolve through the years. Pay interest to those changes, modify your exercises accordingly, and keep ordinary conversation with healthcare specialists to make nicely-knowledgeable choices.

Maintain Optimism and Adaptability: Menopause is a transformative length. Approach it with an open mind, flexibility, and positivity to completely include this lifestyles chapter.

CONCLUDING THOUGHTS ON FLOURISHING DURING MENOPAUSE:

Thriving through menopause extends beyond symptom control—it entails coming into a brand-new lifestyles section with renewed energy, self-assurance, and self-compassion. Each girl's menopausal enjoy is distinct, and finding your course means embracing what suits you best. Remember that this journey isn't always a single event however an ongoing process of evolution, mastering, and personal increase.

As you development, continue to prioritize your properly-being. Trust in your capability to navigate this period with poise, armed with the essential equipment, wisdom, and energy. Here's to flourishing past menopause greeting each day with reason, fitness, and pleasure on this effective new bankruptcy

APPENDIX

Supplementary Materials for Navigating Menopause Successfully
Every female report menopause differently, and the adventure extends beyond analyzing a single manual. To help you in dealing with this existence segment, we've compiled a list of extra assets that offer extra insights, aid, and sensible strategies. Remember, being nicely-knowledgeable empowers you, and gaining access to records and help can transform this transition right into a greater high quality and much less intimidating experience.

1. Suggested Literature

A big range of books on menopause, hormonal health, and common wellness can decorate your knowledge. Here are a few tremendously encouraged titles:

The Wisdom of Menopause by using Christiane Northrup, M.D.: A great guide exploring the physical and emotional shifts for the duration of menopause, providing perspectives on how this period can foster non-public improvement.

Menopause Confidential by Tara Allmen, M.D.: A clean and on hand e book protecting menopausal signs, remedies, and lifestyle recommendation.

The Hormone Cure by using Sara Gottfried, M.D.: Concentrates on natural hormone balancing, providing hints on food plan, lifestyle selections, and supplements that promote hormonal nicely-being.

2. Digital Resources and Support Communities

*   North American Menopause Society (NAMS): A prominent enterprise devoted to advancing ladies fitness through menopause studies and schooling. Their website provides sincere records and resources.

*   International Menopause Society (IMS): An organization presenting a worldwide perspective on menopause and midlife

health, presenting educational content material and study's findings.

Menopause Support Groups: Online communities, together with Facebook groups or health internet site boards, can offer a experience of belonging and shared reviews. Interacting with others going through similar situations can increase feelings of isolation and offer comfort.

3. Nutrition and Fitness Resources

Menopause-Specialized Registered Dietitians: Seeking advice from a dietitian who focuses on girls's fitness and menopause can provide tailor-made dietary steerage.

Exercise Programs for Menopausal Women: Physical pastime is critical for bone health, weight management, and mood regulation during menopause. Many health facilities, studios, and on-line structures offer training tailored to this life stage, which include power training, Pilates, and yoga.

Health and Wellness Tracking Apps: Applications like MyFitnessPal (for nutrition), Headspace (for meditation), and Fitbit (for bodily activity tracking) allow you to track your wellbeing routines and promote consistency.

4. Alternative and Complementary Approaches

Herbal Remedies and Supplements: Certain herbs and supplements, which include black cohosh, nighttime primrose oil, and red clover, are regularly discussed for assuaging menopause signs. Consulting a healthcare provider or licensed herbalist can manual you in selecting secure and powerful options.

Mind-Body Techniques: Meditation, deep respiratory physical games, and practices like mindfulness can assist control stress and enhance emotional nicely-being. Local studios or online systems often provide instructions or tutorials on these techniques.

Acupuncture for Menopausal Symptoms: Some women have discovered acupuncture useful in decreasing hot flashes, tension, and sleep disturbances. Consulting a licensed acupuncturist may additionally offer extra relief alternatives.

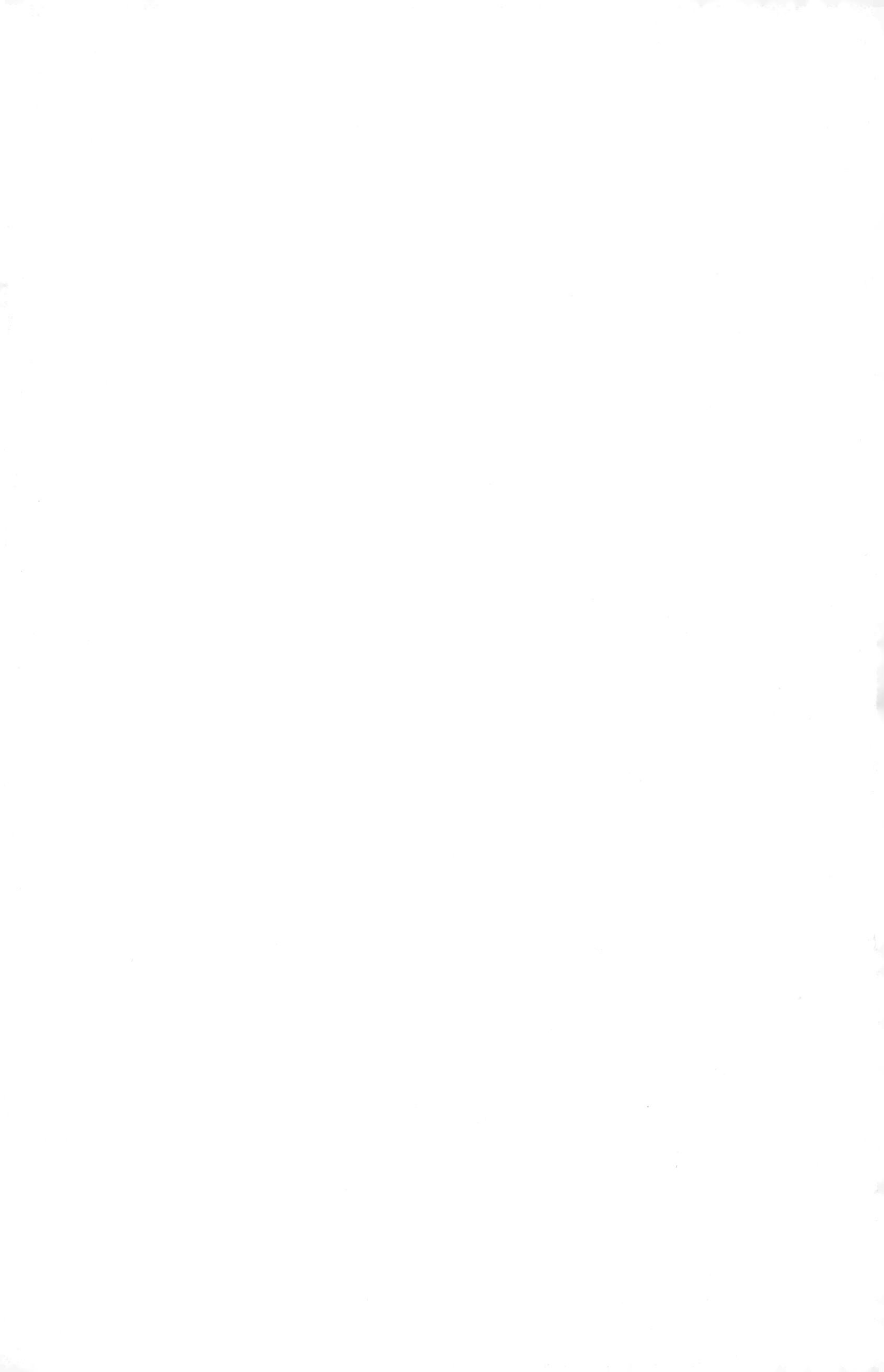